Contents

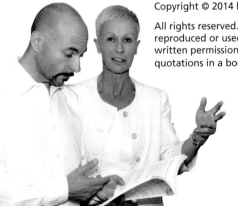

www.elementsofhealth.info

First Publication, 2014

ISBN 978-1-49437-261-3

Green Shoots Publishing
Neubaugasse 4/2/18
1070 Vienna
www.GreenShootsPublishing.com

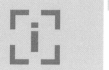

Introduction

What is health? What keeps us fit and alive? What improves our quality of life and keeps us balanced and healthy? Why does one person live to be a 100 and others, like my mother, die at 50 because of cancer? These questions and the mysterious world of body, mind and spirit in their totality touched me deeply when I was young and lead me into the profession of journalism.

That was 20 years ago and since that time I have worked for several important health magazines and publications, doing a lot of intense research, always in the field of health. I spent a long time trying to establish a connection between the truth and scientific evidence.

In my professional research as journalist I pursued healing methods from all corners of the world till I found my most important guideposts, Dr. Ursula Rustler and Peter J Levine. Finally I got the answers I was looking for. I was startled by the difference in their approach and delighted by the results of treatment. In our numerous interviews and conversations I discovered a new world and a new way of thinking about health, myself and the way to approach living.

It is important that this simple and powerful message is available to anyone who wants to find out how to improve their life and health. So I'm delighted to write this introduction and hope as many readers as possible will get the same benefits that I have enjoyed from working with Ursula and Peter.

What is it that you hope or expect to find on the following pages? It is the Elements of Health, the result of the work of two visionaries, experts in their respective fields; Dr Ursula Rustler, one of the few women practitioners of both Western and Oriental medicine, and Peter J Levine holistic pioneer, holistic lifestyle coach and author (The Mechanics of Happiness series).

Their story is one of two skilled practitioners who found and complement each other. Their combined experience covers more than sixty years and the result is a practical vision which provides the keys for maximum health and well-being for anyone – providing they want it. They set themselves the task of creating a practice where easy to implement strategies giving proven results can be applied, demonstrated and taught. An approach that maximises the physical, mental, emotional and spiritual potential of any person; they called this method The Elements of Health (EoH).

I wish you the very best as you read more and discover a new way of thinking about health, yourself and the way you approach living. May you gather as many benefits, improvements and answers from this as I have. I am sure you will.

Evelyne Huber

Vienna 2013

Body   Mind   Feelings   Spirit

The Story of the Elements of Health
Why did we create the Elements of Health?

Many major breakthroughs follow personal experience. The experience itself is often incidental in a sequence that provides a key to unlock greater understanding. In our own story this was absolutely the case, we were both exposed to things that we might not otherwise have chosen to face but whose influence had a dramatic effect upon us as people and the way we viewed our own lives. We thought it would be useful if we explained in our own words some of the reasoning behind the Elements of Health.

Ursula: My brother died of cancer when I was a medical student. That had a huge impact on me. It made me consider my own life differently, particularly what I could do to help others both as a doctor and an individual. Through that experience I discovered that the physical medicine and care available satisfied some but not all the needs of someone who is facing major trauma.

I realised that the approach to health in general is limited. So often we consider health only when it is gone, when we are ill. When a person is ill their concern for their health is acute. When they are well, that same person is, understandably, less urgent about their health. However, the evidence is overwhelming that our lifestyle and the way we take care of ourselves when we are well has a direct influence upon the kinds of illness we become susceptible to. Significantly, people who take good care of themselves spend far less time dealing with the consequences of poor health.

The key to this is your education, not about learning how to earn your way in the world; the education that is needed is a whole life strategy that takes into account all parts of a person's life, not just their physical well-being.

Body   Mind   Feelings   Spirit

We are much greater than the sum of our individual parts. Holism deals with what makes a human being, the whole person, not just their body. A person's spiritual life, feelings or emotional well-being and mental health are just as important as their physical health. What became clear to me was that physicians simply don't have the time to deal with these things; they are so busy repairing what's gone wrong. The best work is done before it gets to that stage, which in no way denigrates the excellent work that medical professionals do. As any doctor will agree, prevention is far better than cure.

Peter: The trace is a long one; I have a background in philosophy, personal growth and development stretching back more than thirty years. The inciting incident happened about ten years ago when I received a diagnosis for a condition that I was told was untreatable, incurable and terminal. I was in my thirties, relatively young, and things like that were not supposed to happen to people my age. It turned my entire world on its head.

I wasn't prepared to accept the diagnosis passively and focused my energies on overcoming the condition. The specialist who worked with me, Professor Chris Day, was able to help with specific information and, by using a range of holistic strategies, I was able to cure the 'incurable' disease.

Because adversity and resistance is part of living, after the initial shock I rolled up my sleeves and got on with it. I refused to passively accept the diagnosis I was given until I had exhausted every possible alternative. People react differently to potentially traumatic news; I realised that my understanding and belief system were about to be seriously and unavoidably tested.

You can't do the same things, think the same thoughts, go on in the same way and expect to get different results. I knew that I had to change if I wanted a different outcome. I needed to look at myself as objectively as possible and implement major

Body　　Mind　　Feelings　　Spirit

change. I understood that if I wanted to bring about inner healing or resolution, I had to fully accept responsibility for myself too.

I had to re-evaluate what was important to me, what actually counted and mattered in my life. Then I had to design a route map that got me from where I was to where I wanted and needed to be. I needed a strategy. First I had to take care of my physical condition, this involved specific forms of diet and exercise that cleansed and purged my system. It moved on to include mental and emotional exercises, meditations and reprogramming.

Over time, I underwent a complete reformation. I am healthier now than at any other time in my adult life. Paradoxically, it was the best thing that could have happened to me because it forced me to confront things that I had avoided and contributed to my condition. I believe fervently in becoming the very thing you say that you want to see in the world. We, as human beings, are generally underachieving because we are not shown how to embrace life fully.

The holistic approach is, beyond doubt, the only authentic path to travel on. To not consider the whole system, body, mind, feelings and spirit, is to miss the point of living. These experiences define us, they make us who we are and they determine the outcomes we get.

The magnificent and spectacularly successful work that Ursula does complements my own perfectly. It was a natural progression to combine what we do and develop a system, a foundation for those wanting to build their own lives, just as we do. Its very simple really, we want people to have access to what we have and enjoy the benefits it can bring to their lives.

We are both passionately committed to maximising health and to personal emancipation, liberation and growth. Authentic development is something that you embody and practise, not just talk about. If you love the idea of development, then become developed; if

Body   Mind   Feelings   Spirit

you love the idea of personal emancipation, become emancipated.

Imagine ...

... somewhere you felt at home, free to explore and discover your own life in a supportive environment. Somewhere that you could drop your guard, and allow yourself to grow, develop and become exactly the person you wanted to be.

... somewhere you could discover how to balance and improve the different aspects of your life. Where the four areas that make up who you are, your Body, Mind, Feelings and Spirit, are explored, explained and expanded in an easy to understand and practical way.

... somewhere the path to authentic happiness, maximum health, fulfilment and satisfaction is clearly laid out; then travelled. Where health is not only about healing you when you're sick but also about living a holistic and healthy lifestyle.

... somewhere safe, informative and educational, filled with discoveries that can help to dramatically improve the quality of your life and save you time and effort trying to do it alone.

Do you want these imaginings to become true? If you do, then this book was written for you.

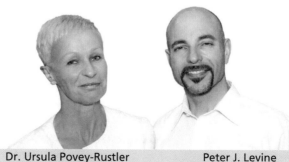

Dr. Ursula Povey-Rustler   Peter J. Levine

Body   Mind   Feelings   Spirit

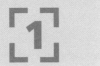

Chapter 1

Most people only think about their health when it's gone.

Health is the balanced relationship between body, mind, feelings and spirit.

Health and wellbeing is as apparent in a person's attitude as it is in their body.

Territorial boundaries exist between physicians, psychologists, therapists and spiritual advisors.

We are conditioned to think of our lives as being compartmentalised, a series of boxes.

We think of our lives from a warped perspective.

Your health depends upon your different domains working seamlessly and smoothly together.

Our systems are fully integrated; we are greater than the sum of our individual parts.

Most people only think about health when it's gone, so the story is often one of regret, anger and negative feelings. Health is commonly considered to be a purely physical thing, which could not be further from the truth. If one thing is certain about health it is the fact that it is determined by the relationship between the four different domains we occupy – our bodies, minds, feelings and spirits.

We have worked with many people over the years and the evidence became overwhelming that health and wellbeing is as apparent in a person's attitude as it is in their body. What then became clear to us was that definite boundaries exist between, for example, physicians, psychologists, therapists and priests. Each attends to their own domain; the physician to your body, the psychologist to your mind, the therapist to your feelings and the spiritual advisor to your spirit.

Because of this territorial division, we are conditioned to think of our lives as being compartmentalised. We tend to think of our different expressions as being separate, distinct and divided. Our bodies are nothing to do with our spirits and our feelings are nothing to do with our minds and so on. It places us in a difficult situation, because we are already considering our lives from a warped perspective. Different groups of people don't 'get' each other, the athletes don't 'get' the psychiatrists who may think that the Zen Buddhists are strange and they all wonder about the therapists!

For you as a person, it isn't like this. Your health is dependent upon exactly the opposite; that your different domains work smoothly, seamlessly together. Your different parts must fit and function co-operatively or become compromised. Our systems are fully integrated; we are greater than the individual sum of our parts. That is holism defined, really. We exist as single beings with multiple expressions.

Body   Mind   Feelings   Spirit

If you consider a machine, something goes wrong with its mechanism and it affects the whole operation unless it is dealt with promptly. If it is not dealt with then it will damage the machine permanently and irrevocably. That's a machine, designed to perform a specific task or operation. You are, in principle, a little like that, the main difference is that you have an innate intelligence that can compensate for difficulties and function at a lesser level. For the world as it is generally, a lesser level 'you' is more than adequate; you can perform various tasks and functions that keeps the world happy and assures you of a place within it.

The next thing to consider is that, just suppose, there were a greater potential for you and your life than merely fulfilling a mechanical type existence. And this is where it gets interesting, because people then start to question the meaning of their mechanical type existence. 'Is this all there is?' they may ask. Then they start to feel unfulfilled, dissatisfied and unhappy. The next stage is that their health is negatively affected.

So we asked ourselves the question, what would happen if someone was aware of this and actively engaged in either prevention or cure of poor health in any domain from a holistic perspective? And we found that this question was not being treated seriously. Experts tend to ignore each other's disciplines so there was no cohesive structure. What was on offer was not substantial and did not lend itself to much scrutiny. Not useful if you're looking for something thorough to help you understand yourself better.

The answer to the question is that, with the right guidance, the person takes control of their own life. Perhaps slowly if they are already unwell, but ultimately they become the one in the driver's seat. They choose, they decide and they take responsibility for their own health and wellbeing. If you are determining the outcomes and the targets then you

We exist as beings with multiple expressions.

You can simply exist within the world – or choose to live your potential for growth, development and wellbeing.

People ask: is this all there is?

Not addressing the important issues in your life has a negative impact upon your health.

Experts tend to ignore each other's disciplines and consequently there was no connected structure or plan.

With the right guidance you can take control of your life.

Body   Mind   Feelings   Spirit

You can define the levels of satisfaction, fulfilment and happiness that you expect and require.

Are you interested in accessing a balanced and informed system to maximise your life potential?

are also defining the levels of satisfaction, fulfilment and happiness. Then we asked ourselves the question, who wouldn't want to be in that position? So ask yourself that same question:

If you could access a balanced and informed system to maximise your life potential in an easy and practical way, surely you would be interested?

And then add to it:

That system places you in control of the health and wellbeing of your body, mind, feelings and spirit; you would have to wonder who wouldn't be interested.

So that was the original premise for the Elements of Health, to create an independent, self determination framework enabling anyone to take control of their own life and make informed decisions about what is best for them. We wanted, more than anything, to change the way you think about your life, to recognise your own power, to become aware of your own capacity and to take the actions necessary to bring about positive and beneficial change in your life.

Now, based on our experience; we know lots of people will have an excuse for not doing what they know is right. Some may think they're too old, others may think they're not healthy enough, some may consider themselves not intelligent enough, others don't think they're spiritually inclined, some don't think they have enough time, and others are just waiting for the right moment... and so on and so on. So our first task is to surround those excuses with reasonable evidence and expose them for what they are, excuses. Our challenge to you is this, who wins, you or the excuse?

And if there are winners and losers in this, what is the prize? Or put another way, what are the benefits to you of saying 'yes' to the Elements of Health?

Body   Mind   Feelings   Spirit

- raised levels of self awareness
- a greater sense of well-being
- a feeling of being reconnected to the bigger picture we are all part of
- learning to accept who you are
- discovering ways to change the things you want to change
- renewed purpose
- tidying up and attending to the important things in your life
- re-opening the door to the simple pleasures in life
- clear direction, objectives and targets that are attainable, practical and do-able
- living a life where qualities such as love, care, patience, understanding, humility, gratitude, respect and joy are consciously practiced
- becoming the person you want to be and living the life you want to live
- becoming relaxed, settled and comfortable with yourself
- exploring and developing your potential
- becoming an asset to yourself, those around you and the human family at large
- learning to live an integrated and more aware life and of course...
- improved physical, mental, emotional and spiritual health

More on these statements - which actually come from clients, patients and seminar attendees - later.

In this book we will explain at an introductory level how to do it, it's easier than you might think, and how it works. To begin, let's draw a simple sketch of the Elements of Health.

The purpose of the EoH is to bring about balance and healing in all areas of your life.

The EoH places you in charge of your life by educating, informing and showing you how to redefine yourself.

We want to help you to improve the quality of your life by empowerment, liberation and the facilitation of positive change.

We want to give you the tools to do the job.

We give you the tools, you do the work, and you get the benefit.

A healthy mind in a healthy body combined with, clearly defined feelings and an active spirit.

Body   *Mind*   *Feelings*   *Spirit*

An Overview

The purpose of the Elements of Health is to bring about balance and healing in all areas of your life, then to promote your living the best possible life. The EoH places you back in charge of your life and its circumstances by educating, informing and showing the way to redefine yourself. The EoH enables you to discover new ways of getting the results you want from the way you live.

The objective of the EoH is to improve the quality of your life by empowerment, liberation and the facilitation of positive change. This may include

- healing
- remedial treatments
- therapeutic support
- coaching
- lifestyle restructuring
- education programmes and
- creating strategies that are solutions focused and person centred, tailored to meet your needs.

Peak physical fitness, a sharp and healthy mind, clearly defined feelings and a healthy spiritual component to your life. These four cornerstones define you, who you are and how you behave. They determine everything about you, so it makes sense that you determine how you want them to be.

At the heart of all things there is balance; a state of harmony and peace which nothing can diminish. It is essential that you have access to that place or state. This is the simple principle that makes the EoH work; bring your Body, Mind, Feelings and Spirit to a state of balance. Are you aware that located within you, perhaps undiscovered, there is a balance point; a place of stillness? A place unaffected by the external challenges of the modern age, when ever increasing speed, epidemics of stress, depression and relentless pressure are exerted upon all of us.

It is this simple principle that makes the EoH work: bring your Body, Mind, Feelings and Spirit to a state of balance.

Increasing speed and information overload place ever greater demands upon our personal resources.

People can't find the elusive work/life balance.

It is about finding an inner state rather than manipulating external circumstances and influences.

The true art of living is to discover your personal balance point so you find authentic happiness,.

Does our materialistic society make us happy?

...quite the opposite.

The way forward is not more of the same, there has to be a different approach, a holistic approach to living

Body   Mind   Feelings   Spirit

People often talk about the work/life balance. They talk about finding that elusive harmony, and then wonder why it doesn't work. The answer is that the balance is not about life and work; it is an inner state that reflects your own internal balance. It is the result of conscious action, not wishful thinking. The four domains, your body, mind, feelings and spirit merge into one another; they combine to make who and what you are. The true art of living is in discovering your personal balance point and applying a strategy that enables authentic happiness, joy and love to flourish in your life.

Materialism has become the dominant characteristic of our age. Material abundance should, theoretically, have resulted in a more contended and happier society. In fact the result has been quite the opposite; more of us than ever before are clinically depressed, medicated and feel disenfranchised. Consider the following conditions, most or all of which are related to the difficulties of coping with the modern world:

- Acid Peptic Disease
- Alcoholism
- Asthma
- Fatigue
- Depression
- Tension Headache
- Hypertension
- Insomnia
- Irritable Bowel Syndrome
- Ischemic Heart Disease
- Psychoneuroses
- Sexual Dysfunction
- Skin diseases like Psoriasis, Lichen planus, Urticaria, Neurodermatitis etc

The chart below gives an indication of just how closely related symptoms and responses are to external and internal causes of stress, anxiety and so on. Somatisation*, or the conversion of psychological distress into physical illness, recognizes that an emotionally distressed patient more often

Body   Mind   Feelings   Spirit

*What is somatisation?

Somatisation is the process by which mental and emotional stresses become physical in the form of psychosomatic illnesses. Some experts believe that, as stresses play on the body, the weakest or most prone system becomes the likely target for somatisation. Others believe the area affected by somatisation has a direct relationship to the nature of the negative thought patterns through mind/body relationships not yet fully understood.

We all have bodies, minds, feelings and spirits. This is what makes us human, yet the connection between the four is all too often missed, ignored or simply unknown.

presents with physical symptoms than psychological complaints. At a more extensive level, the whole person - you, is an interconnected network whose wellbeing is determined by being in a state of balance.

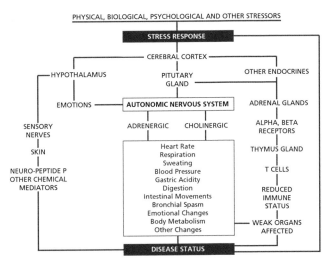

This cocktail of symptoms, causes and effects make many people want to try to change the world. What remains constant, however, is that the only thing you can genuinely change is yourself.

We all have the same basic equipment. We occupy four distinct domains, our bodies, minds, feelings and spirit. We experience things through this fourfold prism, the quintessence of which is being human. Because you are educated according to the requirements of the world, you lack genuine life knowledge. You may be a captain of industry, extremely productive and useful to the world, however this does not mean you are extremely productive and useful to yourself. You may be a successful working mum, wealthy, admired, and famous even, but unhappy, lacking power. You may be a career high flier, your profile may have 'success' stamped all over it but still something is missing; a vital component is lacking that makes worldly success meaningless.

Body   Mind   Feelings   Spirit

You can't change the world – you can only change yourself.

Material abundance doesn't guarantee happiness.

In the absence of genuine life knowledge can lead to an imbalance in Body, Mind, Feelings or Spirit.

The EoH considers you through the four domains and concentrates on restoring balance throughout your entire system.

Some people have a feeling of emptiness inside, feeling that somehow, something is missing.

You may be someone or know people who appear to have everything, the world at their feet, yet beneath that exterior they are desperately unhappy, confused, lost and drifting. And this feeling of lack of control is the ultimate equal opportunity employer. It can occupy men, women, the old, the young, the wealthy, the poor, the employed, the unemployed, single people, married people, gay, straight, divorced or whatever. It doesn't care what colour you are, where you live, how you dress, what job you do, whether you attend a church or a temple, a mosque or a synagogue. It doesn't care if you are a believer or an atheist, agnostic or open to persuasion. You may appear to hold the reins of the world in your hand... yet, something is absent; something vital is missing.

Why is this? Why are people who on the face of it have everything, anxious, unhappy, insecure, depressed and struggling to cope? They do not recognise their own imbalance. EoH has the keys to recognise, become aware of the symptoms and take remedial or preventative action so that your body, mind, feelings and spirit do not become so estranged from one another that they break down in some way.

In the absence of sound guidance or 'genuine life knowledge' we can become easily disoriented. Some parts of our lives, the physical for example, are over indulged while others are neglected. This can be any combination; the mind is over indulged while the feelings are neglected; the emotions unrestrained and dominant and so on. The result of all these combinations is imbalance. When something is imbalanced it is liable to collapse, topple or fall. Critically, this imbalance is directly responsible for much of the difficulty and confusion we experience. If you ignore an imbalance in one of the domains then the whole system is in trouble.

Body   Mind   Feelings   Spirit

The Elements of Health considers you through the four domains – Body, Mind, Feelings, and Spirit. To do anything else is to ignore a fundamental truth of our existence. The approach is disarmingly simple:

EoH helps you

- To recognise
- To become aware
- To understand

EoH enables you

- To heal where necessary
- To restore balance

EoH is an essential support

- To develop
- To refine

This simple process is applied to all of the domains with the objective of bringing about optimum health. No two people experience the same journey but the principles that define the process are the same for all of us. There is no need to endure a situation that keeps you away from living a full and rewarding life; you have the power to choose life.

Body   Mind   Feelings   Spirit

Chapter 2
What are the benefits of the Elements of Health?

What do most people want to achieve?

Wealth beyond their wildest dreams, success, fame, recognition, the greatest love story ever told, significance, truth, no regrets, to make a difference… and the list goes on because it is a subjective list. Of course, we've left off your personal favourite, whatever it might be. What do these things really mean? What gives you the power to chase and achieve your dreams or ambitions? The knotty issue people often gloss over is the question, what price do you actually pay for the outcomes you get? So are you living how you want to live, or are you building castles in the air because you've been told that is what you should want? Think about this carefully, because 'What do I want?' is one of the most potent questions you can ask yourself, and are you prepared to pay the price?

What do we want to achieve?

We want to show you how to achieve maximum health in the four domains of your life.

Think for a moment about what that actually means. Consider the potential improvement that represents in every department of your life. Without holistic health, all the other things are pipe dreams, no more than fantasies.

We want to show you how to do it for yourself without costing you everything you have and not realising it until all your resources have been used. We want you to wake up and exercise the power that you have while you still have the power to do so.

Even to be reading this now means that it's not too late to begin. In fact it's never too late but how often have you heard that being wheeled out as an excuse for doing nothing? Be honest with yourself for a

Are you living the life you want or are you living something else?

If money is the acme of success, what price are you paying for the money that you earn?

The EoH wants to show you how to achieve maximum health in the four domains of your life.

To live an authentic holistic life you need a strategy that is based upon beng in harmony with yourself and the four domains that constitute what you are.

Wake up and live!

It's never too late to begin, but it's already later than you think.

Get rid of the idea that the only criteria for success are material possessions, rank, status and other temporary things.

Be honest with yourself for a moment. What's your excuse? Is that excuse a luxury you can afford?

Body   Mind   Feelings   Spirit

Example excuses:

I'm too old
I'm not intelligent enough
I don't have the time
I'm not fit enough
I'm not the right kind of person
I'm not a team player
I don't believe I can change myself
I'm too set in my ways
I don't have a good educational background
I've heard it all before
I don't trust things that I can't physically hold or touch or see

Good health practices are so well documented it makes almost no sense to mention them. The issue is not one of what they are, rather it is about why people neglect to do them.

Physical health is not something that is a lifestyle choice, it's not a box you tick dependent on whether you're interested or not.

Your mind never stops assimilating new information, learning new things and is always ready to change.

You're never too old to learn.

moment, no-one else can hear you thinking, what's your excuse? Can you afford to have an excuse?

Now let's continue by looking at the benefits of the Elements of Health through the health of the four domains, your Body, Mind, Feelings and Spirit.

Domain One: Your Body

Your body is the greatest resource you have, the foundation upon which everything else is built. To be at a state of maximum health is desirable and achievable. Your future well being and ability to maximise your own potential is dependent upon your physical condition being the best possible.

There is a global problem; people simply don't take good care of themselves. Raised blood pressure leading to increased coronary heart disease, and chronic respiratory conditions are currently pandemic. Worldwide 2.8 million people per year die as a result of being overweight or obese. Being overweight or obese increases the risk of heart attack, ischemic stroke, type 2 diabetes mellitus and some common cancers.

Between 1980 and 2008 worldwide prevalence of obesity almost doubled. By 2008 10% of men and 14% of women (half a billion people) were obese compared with 5% of men and 8% of women in 1980. Source: *World Health Organisation Global Statistics 2012.*

Good health practices are essential to achieve and maintain excellent physical wellbeing. The Elements of Health approach covers everything from physical exercise to dietary intake to personal health strategies created for you and based upon what is best for your current condition and needs.

Physical health has to be an absolute default setting. Taking care of the greatest gift you have ever been given should not be a box that you tick dependent upon whether you're interested or not.
Good physical health is the supreme gift of living,

Body   Mind   Feelings   Spirit

ask anyone who is ill or has poor physical health. It becomes the goal, the objective and the reason for living; good physical health is the key that fits the lock which opens the door to living the best life possible.

Domain Two: Your Mind

It used to be thought that at a certain point you could not learn any thing new. Your mind was, in effect, full. Now we know that this is not the case, it never was, but the myth persisted. Research into synapse formation and development indicates that we can carry on learning until the day we die, at whatever age that may be. This is fantastic news, because it means that mentally you are never too old, and your mind remains dynamic throughout your life.

Once, pioneers were driven to push back the frontiers of unexplored continents, wildernesses, the world's oceans and outer space. The greatest frontier is the same as it ever was: the human mind, human potential and all it is the gateway to.

Mental health is often overlooked because there is no immediately apparent physical evidence of its neglect. However, the principles of good health: regular exercise, healthy diet and taking good care of the system apply to all domains. There are currently enormous problems regarding mental health such as a global crisis in depression, increased dementia in the elderly and substance abuse issues. Stress and its related conditions such as 'burn out' are spiralling out of control, costing billions in financial and human resources.

The World Health Organization (WHO) defines mental health as a 'state of well-being in which every individual realizes his or her own potential, can cope with the normal stresses of life, can work productively and fruitfully, and is able to make a contribution to her or his community'. We are committed to your achieving and surpassing that definition.

Body   Mind   Feelings   Spirit

"One looks back with appreciation to the brilliant teachers, but with gratitude to those who touched our human feelings. The curriculum is so much necessary raw material, but warmth is the vital element for the growing plant and for the soul of the child."
C G Jung

Your emotions are an incredibly powerful force within your life, whether you like it or not.

Your feelings are like a physical landscape. Sometimes, it is barren and rocky with soaring peaks and dramatic valleys.

Sometimes it is a gently flowing and fertile landscape; which one is a better environment to create your feeling home?

"When you start becoming really successful, the demons start to tempt you - the demons of vanity and self importance, drug abuse, the feelings of fraudulence. But, it's also a thrill. That's what I found weird."
Ethan Hawke

"A spiritual person is also in touch with his or her own reality, feelings and thoughts, and the reality of the people around him or her, not projecting on them."
Keith Miller

You have the option to be proactive in your mental health and wellbeing. The EoH works with you not only to achieve optimum mental health but also enables you to embrace and explore the remarkable world that is opened by a healthy mind.

Domain Three: Your Feelings

What do you feel about anything? How fluent are you with your feelings in any given situation and, significantly, are you in control of these feelings? Feeling happy or sad, bright or dull, positive or negative are clearly big influences in how we perceive things. The critical point is this, do you define your feelings or do they define you? Are you familiar with the map of your own emotional landscape and can you navigate it skilfully? Or perhaps you are lost in an intimidating landscape that you didn't even realise you could shape and model according to the needs of your own life?

That's where we start, that's the boot camp. This extends to a level that is increasingly eloquent and fluent, a state where you are the conductor of the symphony being played by your own internal orchestra. The alternative is a painful noise, a cacophony without direction, form or meaning. Where would you rather be?

Your emotions are an incredibly powerful force within your life, whether you like it or not. We are all subject to them, pride, guilt, vanity, embarrassment... the list goes on. They colour our behaviour, decision making, character development and subsequently the outcomes we experience.

Emotional health and wellbeing is predicated by the same principles of exercise, diet and an effective care and maintenance regime that influence the other domains. The process of healing your feelings or emotions takes as its basic premise the restoration of balance or harmony.

Body   Mind   Feelings   Spirit

To achieve the optimal condition, you have to establish equilibrium, order and balance in your feelings. If we build unstable emotional structures they will, when compromised or challenged, fall.

Consider the feeling landscape as if it were a physical landscape. In many instances, it is barren and rocky with soaring peaks and dramatic valleys. It may also be cold and infertile, arid and dry. These are not bountiful places to live, they may be breathtaking but they are not nurturing environments; an occasional visit, maybe, but not the place to build your home.

The alternative is a gently flowing and fertile landscape, one that supports and sustains life easily and generously. This is a more suitable, benign environment to create your home. In your feeling and emotional lives these are the things you have to consider; do you seek stability and order, or are you subjected to chaos and instability?

To achieve the optimal condition, you have to establish equilibrium, order and balance in your feelings. If we build unstable emotional structures they will, when compromised or challenged, topple. The healing art is to recognise what is already there, how it is arranged and to become aware of the likely outcome of such an arrangement. The next stage is to take action; consider reformation and restructuring of the feeling and emotional landscape so that it supports and enriches rather than compromises your experience. This requires objectivity, care and sensitivity, but it is no less than any of us merit whether we are on the road to repair or refinement.

With understanding, patience and those other feelings that represent the finer end of the emotional spectrum, restoration can occur and you are freed of unnecessary baggage. This enables you to engage more fully with the feeling domain, with your own feelings less compromised and enables you to handle a broader spectrum of feeling experience.

Body   Mind   Feelings   Spirit

Domain Four: Your Spirit

"Just as a candle cannot burn without fire, men cannot live without a spiritual life."
Buddha

Your spirit is like a handful of seeds that under the right circumstances may germinate, take root and establish themselves, blossom, bloom and bear fruit.

"The happiness and peace attained by those satisfied by the nectar of spiritual tranquillity is not attained by greedy people restlessly moving here and there."
Chanakya

One of the fundamental requirements of living a fulfilled life is to embrace spiritual fulfilment. The EoH does not take a dogmatic approach to your Spirit but we encourage you to embrace your own spiritual fulfilment, loyal to Creation itself.

[1] Benson, P. L., Roehlkepartain, E. C., & Rude, S. P.
(2003). Spiritual development in childhood and adolescence: Toward a field of inquiry. Applied Developmental Science, 7, 204–212.

The health of your Spirit extends from being free of unnecessary burdens. The evidence gathered by countless human beings in many situations over many years is that the world we live in is a place that tends to burden and constrict the Spirit rather than open it.

Our approach is simple, your Spirit is like a handful of seeds that under the right circumstances may germinate, take root and establish themselves, blossom, bloom and bear fruit. Those right circumstances are a fertile soil, nourishment and energy. Taken as a holistic continuum, your Spirit is attracted and encouraged by the emancipation of its three co-domains, your Body, Mind and Feelings.

Spiritual development is the process of growing the intrinsic human capacity for self-transcendence, in which the self is embedded in something greater than the self, including the sacred. It is the developmental "engine" that propels the search for connectedness, meaning, purpose and contribution.
It is shaped both within and outside of religious traditions, beliefs and practices. [1]

Beyond its recognition, awareness and deciding what action to take, we approach the health of the spirit as a four-fold process:

- Emancipation
- Liberation
- Illumination
- Enlightenment

The health and freedom of your Spirit is a vital cornerstone of what we do, a basic premise that influences the practical considerations of our work.

One of the fundamental requirements of living a fulfilled life is to embrace spiritual fulfilment. We do not take a dogmatic approach to your Spirit and have no particular bias other than a loyalty to Creation itself.

Body   Mind   Feelings   Spirit

"You are not a human being in search of a spiritual experience. You are a spiritual being immersed in a human experience."
Pierre Teilhard de Chardin

We recognise life as a sacred spark. Life itself is the spirit of the universe.

As human beings we represent the conscious part of the universe's expression. Mostly we are sleeping, but the opportunity to wake up is always with us.

Simplicity is the key.

Small things are the fertile soil for the authentic growth of the human spirit.

It is in the many small things that ultimately we lay the platform for authentic human living.

We acknowledge the principle that Creation is the mechanism of the Creator, which is itself the origin of a Spiritual presence that permeates the Universe.

Put simply, we recognise life as a sacred spark. Life itself is the Spirit of the Universe and we, human beings, are a storehouse of dormant potential expressed through the gift of life itself. Our birthright is the potential to explore and refine our condition as individuals, as communities and societies. It starts with you and the decision that you make to embrace and celebrate your life or the excuse that you come up with to exclude yourself from the greatest pageant that ever existed, the gift of life and the extraordinary gift of being human.

Simplicity is the key to allowing the Spirit to bloom. Small things, not grand and expansive gestures, are the tenets of Spiritual growth and regeneration. We focus upon the many small things that constitute growth and development. Small things which subsequently lay the foundations for the four-fold process - Emancipation, Liberation, Illumination, Enlightenment - that is the platform authentic human living rests upon.

A Spirituality footnote

In the years following World War II, culminating in the 1960s and 70s, there was an appetite for new ways to approach living. Central to this search for how to live the best possible life was a renewed hunger to explore spirituality as distinct from organised religion; driven by people like Aldous Huxley, Timothy Leary, Jack Kerouac, Allen Ginsberg and others. To satisfy that hunger, the emergence of secular ad hoc groups such as the beatniks, hippies and the psychedelic movement created a counter culture whose remnants still exist as a miscellany of eastern influenced ventures in most large western cities.

At the same time perhaps even in response, we witnessed a renaissance of orthodox religious

 Body   *Mind*   *Feelings*   *Spirit*

fundamentalism; exemplified by the Islamic Revolution in Iran in 1979 and the politicisation of various Christian sects in the United States. The result of both these developments, faux esoteric spirituality and a climate of intolerance and bigotry, helped to reinforce a negative perception that spirituality is the province of disaffected individuals or groups of isolated radicals who struggle to accept the world as it is. Spirituality was maligned by influential contemporary psychoanalysts, particularly by Sigmund Freud (1961), who referred to "religion as a universal obsessional neurosis," a mere illusion derived from infantile human wishes (The Future of an illusion p. 43). This outcome has been an egregious failing for us all, a distraction that has caused us to lose sight of something intrinsic.

The mendacity of this perception has ushered us into something of a dead end, a road that leads nowhere and has been detrimental to the collective wellbeing of the entire human race. It is important to set these paths aside and redefine spirituality as the legitimate domain that it is; an essential component of each of us. Our spiritual being is as inescapable a fact as our bodies, minds and feelings. Without embracing and celebrating it, our lives are incomplete and therefore unfulfilled.

The EoH seeks to remove the mystique and the veneer of psychobabble from the spiritual domain and replace those mistaken perceptions with the understanding that it is a completely normal - albeit it personal and private - and vital aspect of our lives.

Living a fulfilled, satisfying and happy life

When they work in harmony, what do these four domains offer us? They offer unlimited possibility, the joys of an open mind and an open heart, physical health and well being and the opportunity to become truly emancipated.

Body   Mind   Feelings   Spirit

The EoH says that an open mind and an open heart, physical health and well being lead to emancipation.

Your life counts and is a priceless gift.

The EoH is the place between the ashram and the hospital where we respect each person's individuality, integrity and uniqueness.

The EoH creates balance by equalising the four domains that your life occupies. The principle is holistic, which means that the sum of what you are is greater than the sum of your individual parts. This is called synergy and our lives, when they are aligned and in balance, become synergistically enhanced. The benefits of this are immense, giving you a greater sense of inclusion, well-being and contentment.

Between the ashram and the hospital there has to be a third place; a place that does not focus upon one domain to the exclusion of the others. EoH is that third place; a place that treats each part of the human with equal priority.

The objectives of Elements of Health are:

- To show you how to create happiness and contentment in your own life
- To place you in control of your own life
- To show you how to get the results you want from the way you live
- To empower you to flourish and prosper in your chosen sphere
- To maximise your health and well-being
- To restore your health and well-being where they are absent or diminished.
- To educate and inform you.
- To help you attain satisfaction, fulfilment and happiness. This serves as the platform upon which to build a purposeful, rewarding and meaningful life.
- To facilitate your becoming emancipated, enhanced and enlightened as your personal journey unfolds.
- To empower you to become more useful to yourself, your family, your community and the world at large.
- Collectively, to further develop a global network of like-minded individuals. A kinship and mutuality with others who share the same or similar views of human life and it's potential as you.

Body   Mind   Feelings   Spirit

The benefits of this to you are

- a greater sense of well-being
- improved physical, mental, emotional and spiritual health
- raised levels of self awareness
- a feeling of being reconnected to the bigger picture we are all part of
- learning to accept who you are
- discovering ways to change the things you want to change
- renewed purpose
- tidying up and attending to the important things in your life
- re-opening the door to the simple pleasures in life
- clear direction, objectives and targets that are attainable, practical and do-able
- living a life where qualities such as love, care, patience, understanding, humility, gratitude, respect and joy are consciously practiced
- becoming the person you want to be and living the life you want to live
- becoming relaxed, settled and comfortable with yourself
- exploring and developing your potential
- becoming an asset to yourself, those around you and the human family at large
- learning to live an integrated and more aware life
- living a holistically improved life in the physical, mental, emotional and spiritual domains

These may seem like big claims; and they are. However, these are all statements that have been made by our patients, clients, and seminar attendees – people who have experienced the Elements of Health and our work. That work being the marriage of more than 60 years study, practice and research by two renowned authorities in the field of health, growth and wellness.

 Body   Mind   Feelings   Spirit

The common theme uniting this endeavour has been our pursuit of what offers the best and most effective results in living an authentic and meaningful life. What, precisely, is it that delivers the greatest and most beneficial return to you as an individual in exchange for the investment of your resources; your time, effort and energy?

What makes the Elements of Health outstanding?

It combines the four disciplines of the
Physician
Psychologist
Psychiatrist
Spiritual adviser

to create a single holistic result.

 Body   *Mind*    *Feelings*   *Spirit*

Chapter 3
How does it work?

The Assessment

How healthy are you to begin with?

Four incisive questionnaires.

Status report

Overview and personal recommendations

Health Status Index

Body Mind Feelings Spirit Continuum

The Elements of Health works simply. First you are assessed, detailed below, and a feedback report is prepared to locate you precisely within the EoH criteria. This is followed by individual coaching sessions, therapeutic sessions, personal support and back-up; and the fulfilment of the 144 exercises of the rebalancing programme. Because you are dynamic, increasingly so once you begin to assert yourself, the whole assessment process is a moving diagram, a record of your change and progress.

The Elements of Health is composed of conventional health assessment methods, Traditional Chinese Medicine (TCM), cutting edge developments in the health, maintenance and well being of the Mind, the Feelings and proven practices in the liberation of the vital inner life force. The combination of these various diverse disciplines creates a unique platform creating awareness, stability and the ideal situation in which to celebrate and embrace your life.

You stand at the centre of a matrix of possibilities, a superhighway of influences which need to be sorted out and tidied up. Over time they have suffered from neglect most often brought about by simple lack of awareness. If you do not know something is there, it is difficult to take care of. The sucker punch is that just because you don't know it's there doesn't mean that it has no influence upon your life, health status and wellbeing. You need to be woken up to a whole universe of influences whose existence has huge implications for your life.

▶ *Body*　　▶ *Mind*　　▶ *Feelings*　　▶ *Spirit*

The Assessment

The initial assessment involves a thorough clinical examination, physical health check and the completion of questionnaires regarding the four domains.

After this you are presented with a status report that reflects where you are Physically, Mentally, Emotionally and Spiritually. The report offers an overview and personal recommendations within the concluding commentary that is totally unique to you and your circumstances. The report alone is an outstanding resource and reference point.

Each area and each question answered is graded individually according to a Health Status Index (HSI). The four domains are known as the BMFS Continuum and your scores are matched to the HSI within the Continuum.

Seven Levels of Health

1. Regeneration
2. Optimal
3. Progressive
4. Stability
5. Misuse
6. Atrophy
7. Premature Degeneration

Regeneration – Degeneration Cycle

You will benefit from the whole process and experience all-round improvement.

Continuum showing »
HSI scores

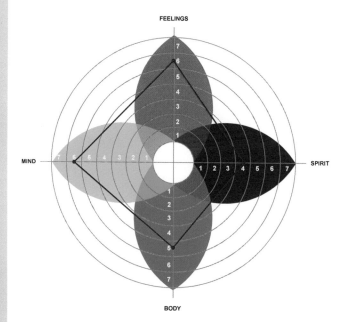

Body   Mind   Feelings   Spirit

The HSI acknowledges seven levels of health:

1. Regeneration
This is when the systems are performing at a higher level and pushing back the boundaries of current capacity.

2. Optimal
This is when the systems are functioning at their peak level.

3. Progressive
Progressive health is when the systems are improving on their current condition as a result of correct maintenance, input and care.

4. Stability
Stability is when the systems are functioning effectively and according to their purpose. In this condition overall health and wellbeing is stable and functioning cohesively.

5. Misuse
When the systems are not employed for purposes that do not serve the integrity and wellbeing of the whole it leads to misuse. Misuse arises from the improper usage of any system within the four domains.

6. Atrophy
This is when the system is heading into decline because of lack of use. Lack of appropriate exercise and maintenance create the conditions of atrophy or wasting away of the system. This is characterised by gradual decline in effectiveness or vigour.

7. Premature Degeneration
This is when the basic qualities of the system have lost their integrity and are in a state of decline not relative to external conditions such as natural ageing. The process is occurring before time, prematurely, and is preventing the system from functioning normally.

This is called the Degeneration-Regeneration (DR) cycle.

Body   Mind   Feelings   Spirit

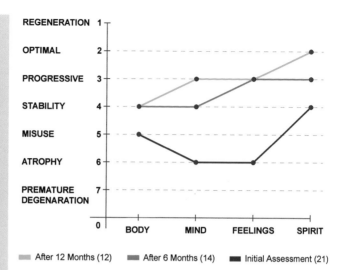

REGENERATION 1
OPTIMAL 2
PROGRESSIVE 3
STABILITY 4
MISUSE 5
ATROPHY 6
PREMATURE DEGENARATION 7
0

BODY   MIND   FEELINGS   SPIRIT

The Health Status Index »

After 12 Months (12)   After 6 Months (14)   Initial Assessment (21)

In the Assessment, your objective is to score the lowest number possible (4) – closest to best possible health.

A higher score indicates that you are further from best possible health.

Each of the seven levels in the Degeneration-Regeneration cycle has five levels or stations:

Regeneration
Renaissance
Reconnection
Rebalance
Repair

Each of the domains has a location on the Degeneration - Regeneration cycle corresponding to its mean level of health. Numerically the objective is to achieve the lowest score possible (4) while the highest numeric value (28) indicates the furthest from best possible health.

The journey to best possible health is progressive and, like any unfolding appearance, has different stages or stations along the way. Each of the locations in the D-R Cycle has its own five level progression status, just like a root system:

1. Regeneration   2. Renaissance
3. Reconnection   4. Rebalance
5. Repair

The resulting matrix is composed of:
Four Domains (Body Mind Feeling Spirit Continuum or the Continuum),
Seven Levels (The Degeneration – Regeneration Cycle),
Five Stages to each of the seven levels.
This forms the dynamic system which is both an assessment tool and a personal mirror.

Your body, mind, feelings and spirit are, at any given time, in a process of states ranging from Premature

Body   Mind   Feelings   Spirit

Degeneration to Regeneration. Each of them operates at different speeds, the body being slowest and the spirit quickest. The different states can be as changing and dynamic as the notes in a piece of music. Your body changes state relatively slowly, but your feelings may move up and down within seconds. The object of the EoH process is to narrow the range between highs and lows while progressing upwards in pursuit of the objective of achieving a state of holistic balance between the four domains. At this point you are able to tap into resources that you may not even be aware you have.

While making this journey the various reflective tools and exercises in the EoH locate you in areas whose improvement will benefit each of the domains.

For example, there may be clear indications that your mind is in a state of atrophy and needs to reconnect to energies that can reinvigorate it. There is a specific exercise concerning this which will be recommended to you. Just so with any of the 144 locations in the matrix; there is a practice or an exercise relevant to each one.

144 specific exercises dealing with different aspects of your Body Mind Feelings and Spirit

The journey from where you are to where you want to be

Simple, practical steps along the road of your progression

The Chart »
of 144 Exercises

Body   Mind   Feelings   Spirit

Each one of the 144 points on the chart has practical exercises, strategies and commentaries relating to it that you can study, practice, engage with and discuss with your personal coach/mentor/strategist.

The progress chart also exists as a 3D topography called The Four Hills which describes your status in an additional graphic form.

„The Four Hills" »
Your personal
Topography

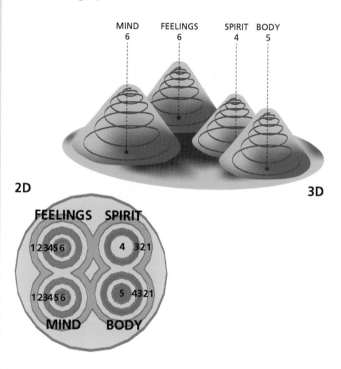

The assessment process is undertaken periodically and allows you to make comparisons between where you were and where you are. The objective is uniform development; progressive development within the four domains in a sustained manner. Over time the **Health Status Index, the Four Hills** and the 144 point **Loom of Reference** becomes a moving diagram recording your own life and the journey you are undertaking. It becomes an invaluable and personal inventory of your development and the progress you are making. It highlights areas of work to focus upon and anything that needs attention.

Body   Mind   Feelings   Spirit

The Practical Exercises

Each of the domains has a sequence of 36 progressive exercises, totalling 144. The exercises define the necessary progressive states that exist on the four pathways along which you travel in order to reach the objective of holistic balance between the four domains. This is defined by a free and unhindered flow of energy throughout your entire system.

The purpose of the exercises is to provide you with a practical foundation upon which to develop greater self awareness and understanding. The exercises include activities, contemplations, strategies, sequences and methods appropriate to each of the four domains. They are designed to cause in you the states within the Pentar of Repair, Rebalance, Reconnection, Renaissance and Regeneration for each of the seven levels within the Degeneration -Regeneration Cycle

Following the initial assessment you will be advised which of the exercises are most appropriate for you based upon the report's findings. This is individual, different for each person and focuses upon the areas needing attention. There are different levels of perception to each exercise and the complete cycle of exercises can be undertaken by you if that is what you want. Alternatively you can choose to do the exercises that take you to a specific level such as stability.

Upon completion of each sequence there is an acknowledgement ceremony of the personal journey you have undertaken and a token is presented to you in recognition of your endeavour.

There is no time frame to the exercises and you may repeat the same exercise many times to extract the vitamin content within it. Some of the exercises will become practices that you carry on for the rest of your life simply because they make you feel good.

[4]

Chapter 4
The relationship between the four domains

The four domains of Body, Mind, Feelings and Spirit merge into one another

The four are the media through which you experience your life

You are the combined result of the actions of all four domains

A healthy body is the most basic requirement for each of us

Theorists, philosophers and great thinkers are all agreed on one thing: You become what you think about

Feelings or emotions are what we experience on an almost continuous basis. Feelings also describe experiences, other than the physical sensation of touch, such as "a feeling of warmth".

Whatever position you take on it, there is indisputably a non material dimension to human existence

To not consider your life as the marriage between four very different but equal parts is to exclude yourself from a truly authentic understanding of whom and what you are.

We are individually unique, but united by a common expression – our Body, Mind, Feelings and Spirit.

The four domains of Body, Mind, Feelings and Spirit are a continuum which means that they merge into one another. They are not separate though their character is different. They occupy the same space, that same space can be more accurately called you. The four are the media through which you experience your life: you have a physical form, you have thoughts, you have feelings and you have a spiritual component to your life. You are the quintessence or combined result of the actions of all four domains.

This interaction is a process, a transference of energy; your health and wellbeing is characterised by the state of this flow of energy. A free and uninterrupted flow characterises optimal health; blockages, hindrances, and stagnation characterise poor health and wellbeing. The relationship between your domains is ideally one of free flow which invigorates, vitalises and energises you.

Let's consider the four domains individually:

Body

A healthy body is the most basic requirement for each of us. We understand that this means different things to different people. Health is a relative state, dependent upon where you're looking from. We place care of the body and meeting its needs as central to enabling you to live the best possible life. In all that we do, we recognise that each individual moves at their own pace, the journey to achieving or maintaining physical health is different for each of us; what matters is that it begins.

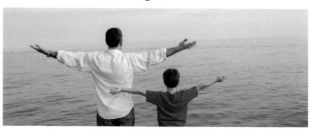

🞂 Body   🞂 Mind   🞂 Feelings   🞂 Spirit

The human body is the most complex piece of equipment. We take the position that rather than being an entitlement and circumstantial to the fact of living, the body is actually a gift, the greatest gift that any of us has ever been given. We each have a duty of care as custodians of a most incredible organism whose sole purpose is to allow you to function effectively within your time here.

Initially, we consider the body to be a mechanism, a highly refined piece of machinery. It requires the kind of care that any piece of precision equipment does. It functions according to its setting, the input we feed it, the smooth flow of its processes and the way that we maintain it.

At the basic level, this involves:

- Awareness
- Diet
- Exercise
- Healing
- Knowing the specifications of the design

Being healthy is the desirable state for each of us, and it is an achievable state. Learning to understand your body and its needs is a simple but essential process. Our approach to living the best life is defined by simple and proven practices that enable you to develop a thorough dialogue with your body. Seeing your life as a holistic partnership between the different domains you occupy and acknowledging that the best outcomes are founded upon the uninterrupted flow of energy between those domains.

It is only when you see your body and your whole life in this context that you can begin to maximise your capacity to live a fulfilled and purposeful life. Balance between the different components gives you access to fulfilment, satisfaction and purpose.

Body   Mind   Feelings   Spirit

Mind

Theorists argue about many things, there is, however, one thing that they all agree on and that is, you become what you think about.

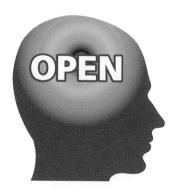

Philosophers and thinkers have found themselves wrestling with the seemingly intractable issue of what they call the 'Mind Body Problem'. In this endeavour, they have struggled to come to terms with and understand the character and nature of thought, the workings of the mind and the way that influences our perception of our environment. This reaches out from our innermost thoughts, fears, concerns, anxieties, hopes and dreams to the societies we construct, the world we live in and the direction that our lives inevitably take.

Unlike your Body, your Mind is not located in the physical domain so it requires a more delicate touch in appreciating and developing a strategy for managing and supporting effectively. Your mind is, in principle at least, like your body - it requires maintenance, the correct input and exercise in order to stay healthy and achieve maximal efficiency. If we take the methods described earlier -

- Awareness
- Diet
- Exercise
- Healing
- Knowing the specifications of the design

- when considering the well-being of your body and apply them to your mind, a distinct pattern begins to emerge concerning taking care of and paying attention to your Mind's wellbeing.

Body   Mind   Feelings   Spirit

Feelings

Perception of the physical world does not necessarily result in a universal reaction among receivers, but varies depending on your tendency to handle the situation, how the situation relates to your past experiences, and any number of other factors. Feelings are a state of consciousness, such as that resulting from emotions, sentiments or desires.

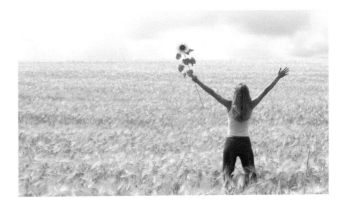

Feelings or emotions are what we experience on an almost continuous basis.

The word was first used to describe the physical sensation of touch through either experience or perception. Feelings also describe experiences, other than the physical sensation of touch, such as "a feeling of warmth". In psychology, the word is usually reserved for the conscious subjective experience of emotion.

We experience our own feelings but also experience the feelings of others. We see, for example, if a person is happy or sad and that has an effect upon our own state. If we see a person or an animal in pain, we may want to ease that pain and bring about a cessation of what we perceive as suffering. If we see someone experiencing joy, we may wish to encourage and support that and experience the feeling of shared joy ourselves.

 Body   Mind   Feelings   Spirit

These are indications of how we experience feelings; they act as intermediaries between the world and ourselves. The awe we feel in the presence of a vast natural occurrence such as mountains, the ocean or a starry sky. The fascination we experience watching a passion-flower open or a colony of ants carrying treasures back to their nest. These experiences inform our awareness and understanding. It is the way things seem to us, a subjective thread that weaves our diverse experiences into a single cohesive fabric. These can be anything from the pain of a headache, the taste of wine, the experience of taking a recreational drug, to the palette of colours in an evening sky.

Our world is an individual and subjective place, unique to us alone. We see things as they are for us, not as they are for others. Central to the appreciation of feelings and emotions in EoH is the notion that even though something seems a particular way to you that may not necessarily be how it is. When we understand this simple core notion, it enables us to handle our own feelings more articulately and with greater skill.

To experience your feelings cleanly, crisply and with a free flow of energy is a great liberation. This can be achieved through the implementation of the methods named in the previous domains of your body and your mind.

Spirit

There are many paths leading to this one absolute.

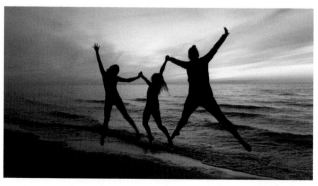

Body   Mind   Feelings   Spirit

Whichever one you take, there is indisputably a non material dimension to human existence. Apparently separate but having synchronicity with the physical world. This often presents as difficult to explore because it can seem enigmatic, mysterious and puzzling.

Our experience of life is so defined by the physical world that the bridge between different states of being can appear elusive. Debates have raged for centuries concerning the nature and even the existence of the Soul, the Spirit, the Divine Spark and numerous other names it has been given.

Such a foundational issue of our lives has, sadly, become clouded by the guerrilla warfare being waged by the scientific and religious communities. Each side blinded to anything other than their own beliefs.

Clearly all the evidence that can be gathered is relevant. This evidence informs our understanding, whether it comes from scientific discovery or from the transcendent sphere of human experience. Everything, when viewed neutrally, offers clues to the nature of whom and what we are.

We champion what is best in human nature and what is possible when humans apply themselves unconditionally. The desire to create and to appreciate beauty, to be a part of something magnificent; these are all symptoms of that essential quality that is intrinsically human. This is magnified by acknowledging the fact of our spiritual being.

It is not possible to understand the character of human life without considering the energising spark within each of us. Our concern is facilitating the emancipation and unfolding of that which lies dormant within.

For us, this position is not theoretical. Evidence gathered over decades has persuaded us conclusively that human life is a spiritual affair with a physical dimension just as much as it is a physical affair with a

Body   Mind   Feelings   Spirit

spiritual dimension. We exist as the condensation of a life force that is no different to the energy that drives the Universe. It is of the same character and is imbued with the same urgencies.

Yet again, when you address your Spiritual domain as you address its three companions -

- Awareness
- Diet
- Exercise
- Healing
- Knowing the specifications of the design

- the increased health, wellbeing and emancipation of the domain will follow.

EOH is independent of any theological or doctrinal influence; our allegiance is to the Universe itself and that which brought it into being. Because of that we are free to explore greater awareness of the holistic character of our lives unhindered by dogma or restriction.

Without a fully engaged spiritual dimension to your life, you cannot be fulfilled, satisfied and complete.

The Four Together

The BMFS Continuum or the Tetrad represents a dynamic system of exchange and information processing. To thoroughly understand, appreciate and fulfil your own potential requires their activation and interaction. Your life is not static, it is constantly changing and you have the potential to personally evolve, to become better than you already are. The Elements of Health is a launch pad into consciously embracing that dynamic state; you can begin to determine exactly how that will happen and the direction you want to go in. When you reposition yourself in the driving seat, you begin to take control of your own life.

That is the promise of the EoH, if not the promise of living altogether, to take control of your own life. To rescue yourself from the difficulties and challenges living in the modern world presents us with. It represents the change from being carried along on the currents of the day to setting a course for a destination of your choosing. The system and the method is the way to make that desire a reality, to turn the promise of living into your way of living and to reap the benefits this brings.

Body   Mind   Feelings   Spirit

Body   Mind   Feelings   Spirit

CPSIA information can be obtained
at www.ICGtesting.com
Printed in the USA
LVIC04n2146280914
406301LV00002B/3